Patient Guide to Semen Analysis

Patient Guide to Semen Analysis

Rajasingam Sivaperagasm Jeyendran, Ph.D.

iUniverse, Inc.
New York Lincoln Shanghai

Patient Guide to Semen Analysis

iUniverse, Inc.

For information address:
iUniverse, Inc.
2021 Pine Lake Road, Suite 100
Lincoln, NE 68512
www.iuniverse.com

ISBN: 0-595-27964-3

Printed in the United States of America

Contents

Preface vii

Summary xi

Author's Disclaimer xiii

Introduction xv

The Male Reproductive System: An Overview 1

Semen Analysis: The Process 16

Conclusion 33

Terminology 35

Definitions & Acronyms 37

About the Author 39

Preface

Your semen analysis can get complicated, and your results, confusing. *Patient Guide to Semen Analysis* has been written for you, the patient, so you can feel more comfortable and fully understand a sometimes confusing, perhaps intimidating, procedure.

Dr. Jeyendran, who has been working directly in this field for over twenty years, feels that an inquisitive and properly informed patient makes the entire fertility management process easier for everyone involved. By knowing exactly what's involved during each step of the process, you and your partner will feel self-assured and more relaxed throughout your fertility treatment regimen.

This guidebook is a simplified, easy-to-read version of Dr. Jeyendran's clinical manual for semen analysis interpretation. *Patient Guide to Semen Analysis* is presented in an accessible and handy "Question & Answer" format, written with you and your needs in mind: No prior medical education or experience is necessary. Several jokes and cartoons have also been added to lighten the reading and shed a humorous light on a sometimes intimidating subject.

If you have any more questions after reading this booklet, feel free to contact the doctor himself. He'll be pleased to answer your inquiries, and even incorporate your various comments and observations into a new edition.

Happy reading, and may your fertility treatment prove successful!

Acknowledgment

The author thanks Michael Spitz for editorial assistance.

Summary

Patient Guide to Semen Analysis is a guidebook designed to help illustrate how this whole process works. This guide describes what your results actually mean, and how these results are related to certain problems you might be having. Should your clinician suggest any form of therapy or treatment, Dr. J.'s book will help explain how these conclusions were reached, and what they might be able to do for you and your partner.

Without a thorough semen analysis and proper interpretation, an otherwise successful pregnancy might be delayed or even neglected.

Author's Disclaimer

While reading this book, please note that some of the author's opinions may not be shared by all other professionals, and therefore should be used only as a constructive guide for understanding your test results.

Importantly, you are advised to follow the recommendation of your own physician. And remember, semen analysis interpretation and physician recommendation is also based on *your partner's* fertility status.

HATS OFF TO THE "HAPPY SPERM"

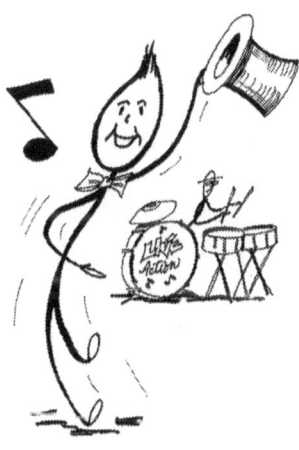

Introduction

"Why should my semen be analyzed?"

These four reasons are typically why a patient will require a semen analysis. One or several of these factors may be relevant for you and your partner's fertility treatment program:

- **Diagnosis and Problem Solving**

  If you and your partner are encountering difficulties having a child, don't worry: You have plenty of company, and should not feel in any way singled-out or ashamed. In truth, fertility problems plague 1-out-of-8 couples of reproductive age in the United States (which is more than 10% of all couples wanting to conceive!).

  Medical scientists estimate that almost half of such fertility issues stem from some problem with *semen quality*. In other words, something about your semen might be making fertilization of your partner (what we'd call, simply, "pregnancy") difficult.

  Conducting a semen analysis is the first step toward diagnosing and hopefully solving any problems you might be having with your semen quality. A semen analysis can also reveal if your semen is actually quite normal, in which case the fertility problem stems from your partner.

  As you'll soon discover, however, the distinction between "normal" and "abnormal"semen is often very subtle and ambiguous. Such an underlying conceptual confusion only heightens the importance of a thorough and thoroughly understood semen analysis.

- **Cryopreservation**

  If, on the other hand, you are about to freeze, or *cryopreserve* your semen for any one of a number of reasons. A preliminary semen analysis is extremely important to help maximize your semen quality before your sperm are frozen for an indefinite period of time.

- **Surgery**

  Semen analysis is also routinely conducted before and after various surgical procedures on the male reproductive system, including vasectomy (male birth control through surgery), and vasovasostomy (corrective surgery).

- **Assisted Reproduction**

  Semen Analysis is also routinely conducted before any assisted reproductive procedure, including artificial insemination and in vitro fertilization.

"What is 'semen analysis'"?

Semen analysis, by definition and not surprisingly, consists of various tests to measure the quality of your semen. These tests are designed to *evaluate* your semen quality, *diagnose* any problems, and offer a *solution*.

Specifically:

- **Evaluation**

  Essentially, semen analysis is a laboratory procedure designed to evaluate the overall quality of your semen.

  You simply want to know: "Is my semen fertile?" The laboratory therefore has to test, interpret the results and then give you an answer: "Yes," "no," or "somewhere in between."

- **Diagnosis**

  Should your semen in any way test as unusual, finding out exactly *what* might be wrong (conducting a preliminary "diagnosis") is next.

  You will want to know: "What is wrong with my semen?" And hopefully the laboratory can then respond: "This," "that," or "something else."

- **Solution**

  After generating these analysis results, the clinician can then decide what, if anything, can be done to *improve* your semen quality.

  In some cases, your semen quality might be affected by certain problems with your reproductive system. A semen analysis can often reveal such problems, and even offer suggestions for their correction, including medical treatments and surgery.

Other instances might simply require a slight change in habit, or even lifestyle. Your job might place you in an environment detrimental to your semen quality, or diet supplementation might be suggested by your clinician. Hormonal therapy might even be offered to help improve semen quality in some instances.

- **Enhancement**

  A practical and proven method for improving sperm quality is *sperm processing*, where samples of your semen are processed in various ways in the laboratory. Sperm processing, in fact, is a vital part of the assisted reproductive process, and can greatly maximize outcome.

  Consequently, semen analysis is routinely performed before such procedures as intrauterine insemination ("IUI") and in vitro fertilization ("IVF"). Semen can also be processed before cryopreservation to help ensure reproductive success after thawing.

  Sperm processing can also help improve your sperm should you be undergoing chemotherapy or any other treatments or ailments that might impair your sperm quality. These enhancement techniques can then hopefully enable your sperm to be successfully used at some time in the future.

"What about my partner? Shouldn't she be tested, too?"

It certainly takes two to tango, especially when fertilization is involved! However, analyzing your semen is much easier and cost effective than conducting initial fertility tests on your female partner.

Acquiring your semen is usually relatively easy. And improving your semen, if that would prove necessary, is often accomplished entirely through laboratory work. Should any problems be found with your reproductive system, most corrective therapies, including surgeries, can be done with relative ease.

In contrast, diagnostic work on your female partner is often intrusive, difficult and expensive. And since close to half of all fertility problems stem from the male, such costly and complicated diagnostic work on your partner might in the long run prove completely unnecessary.

The smart and responsible first step of any fertility treatment method is checking the male out—that means you. If any problems are found, they should be tackled. Meanwhile, your partner should also be evaluated. Note that since performing your partners' tests can be invasive and costly, your test should be done first.

"Old News"

After about half an hour, a man returned rather exasperated from the collection room at the fertility clinic.

"What's the matter?" asked his female partner, greeting him.

"This semen analysis business is hard work!" he replied. "I hope you appreciate what I'm doing for you!"

"Appeciate!" exclaimed the woman, outraged. "You have no idea how easy your part is! Here I am, subjected to an hour-long, internal examination with exotic instrumentation, and all *you* have to do is go into a room, read dirty magazines, and jerk-off into a cup!"

"Sure," her partner responded, non-chalantly. "But those magazines were so out of date!"

"How does semen analysis work?"

- **Semen**

  "Semen," or the male ejaculate, basically consists of the male gene-carrying cell ("sperm") and various secretions designed to nourish and protect it ("seminal plasma").

- **Analysis**

  Semen analysis involves laboratory procedures designed to test these various parts of your semen. Since "a chain is only as strong as its weakest link," the relative healthiness of each semen component contributes to the overall fertilization capacity of your semen.

  These semen tests measure and evaluate many different attributes of your semen, including general appearance, color, amount, activity and other factors.

  As we'll see, some of these properties might prove vitally important for healthy sperm, while others remain surprisingly irrelevant to the fertilization potential of your semen.

- **Sperm**

  The fundamental component of your semen, however, is *sperm*. Your sperm is the semen component that carries all your genetic information; your sperm is the cell that fertilizes your partner's egg.

  Evaluating male fertility is what a successful semen analysis is all about. Therefore, such an analysis should be as simple as clinically determining the quality of your sperm.

  Right?

  Wrong.

- **Sperm Variability**

  All other factors being equal, sperm vary greatly in their quantity and quality. And since all it takes for fertilization to occur is one healthy sperm to get to an egg, such a statistical analysis of millions upon millions of sperm in any given sample can really make even accomplished technicians scratch their chins.

  In other words, the question then becomes: "Can we safely say that this whole sample is actually fertile, or not?" After all, what does it mean for a sample of millions of individual sperm to be "fertile"?

  SIZE DOESN'T MATTER

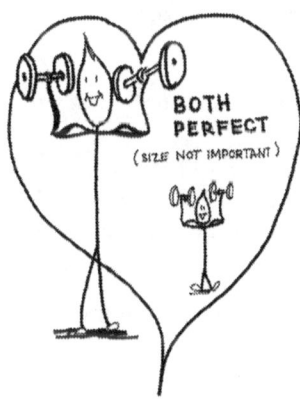

- **"A Perfectly Simple Test"—In Theory**

Here's one idea for a way of finding out if your sperm are capable of getting your partner pregnant: Actually try to fertilize an egg in the laboratory.

Under ideal scientific conditions, your sperm could be prepared to fertilize an egg in the laboratory, under what are called "test tube" or *in vitro*, circumstances. These artificially created laboratory conditions mimic the atmosphere and chemical environment of your partner's reproductive system.

Unfortunately, such a procedure is technically difficult and morally complicated, and won't help diagnose what, if anything, might be wrong with your sperm if the egg *doesn't* get fertilized.

So what can be done?

- **"An Imperfectly Complicated Test"—In Practice**

As a practical and reliable substitute, a number of different tests have been developed to indirectly evaluate the relative fertilitization capacity of your sperm.

The ability of your sperm to potentially fertilize an egg depends on the status of a number of different *sperm variables*. These variables are various physical and behavioral qualities of your sperm.

These sperm variables are then individually measured in the laboratory with certain clinical procedures. When taken together, these tests amount to what is simply called a "semen analysis."

In greater detail, then, the numerous *sperm variables* measured by a typical semen analysis include:

- *Sperm Concentration*
  The actual number of sperm in your ejaculate

- *Sperm Motility*
  The relative ease by which your sperm move through liquids

- *Sperm Morphology*
  Your sperm cells' shape and physical condition

"So what's so complicated?"

Once your semen is analyzed, your sperm evaluated, and all lab results are in, the answer to the basic question "Can my semen make my partner pregnant?" actually becomes much more complicated than you might think.

Unlike other medical tests you might be familiar with, the results of a semen analysis are rarely, if ever, conclusive. In fact, semen analyses do not account for how your sperm may travel through the female reproductive tract to reach the egg. Since such a journey is obviously essential for pregnancy to occur, your semen analysis does not provide all information necessary to judge your sperm as conclusively "fertile" or "infertile".

"Why? I'm either 'fertile' or 'infertile', right?"

No, and for a number of reasons, including:

- **Variation**

  The first clue is that large variations can (and normally do) occur in your results, even between samples taken consecutively.

  For example, the number of sperm measured in any given sample can vary by as much as 200% from the results of your very next sample.

  Such variation isn't surprising, either, when you consider that literally millions of sperm are released in any given ejaculation. With so many sperm released, and each sperm having its own unique construction, the measurement of any given sperm variable seems a rough estimate at best.

- **Definitions**

  Since a clear cut difference does not exist between what is considered "normal" and "abnormal", "fertile" and "infertile", these definitions are highly subjective.

  In other words, where do you set the boundary between what's considered "healthy" and "unhealthy" semen?

- **Sperm Lottery**

  Think about it: All that's necessary for pregnancy is ONE relatively healthy and extraordinarily lucky sperm to get to and penetrate your partner's egg.

Consequently, even if your sperm quality is very poor overall, one sperm out of millions, under a rare set of conditions, might "get lucky" and get your partner pregnant.

Indeed, examples of such "surprise" conceptions coming from men with otherwise poor sperm quality are more common than you might imagine (though much less common than what we would all like). Similarly, if your sample contains very few good sperm, one of these may get lucky, and enable you to fertilize your partner's egg.

THE FERTILE INFERTILE COUPLE: "SURPRISE SURPRISE!"

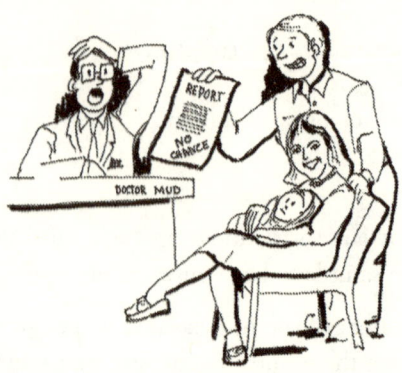

"Can't my partner and I just keep trying? Why even bother with analysis?"

A proper semen analysis, combined with good interpretation and follow-up, can *astronomically* help increase your chances of making your partner pregnant. And in some cases, a proper semen analysis might reveal a fertilization potential of zero or near-zero, suggesting various laboratory or surgical procedures to help overcome a specific physiological problem.

Remember, a proper semen analysis will let you know if your semen is fertile, and to what extent. Hopefully, a properly conducted analysis will increase that likelihood with the help of clinical techniques and perhaps therapies.

The Male Reproductive System: An Overview

Since most problems involving male fertility directly involve the male reproductive system, a broad overview of male physiology and function can greatly facilitate your understanding of the entire therapy process.

"How does the male reproductive system work?"

- **One Early Idea**

  The ancient Greek philosopher Hippocrates theorized that semen was created in the brain and spinal column, then secreted through the blood.

  Obviously, medical science has come a long way since those early times, when the expression "having sex on the brain" was perhaps taken somewhat more literally.

- **Aristotle Over Easy**

  An even more respected ancient, Aristotle, who influenced scientific thinking through the Middle Ages, concluded that the human female had nothing to do with reproduction.

  He felt that since a man's semen could be seen, while the female's egg, unlike a chicken's, remained invisible, that the human egg was therefore non-existent.

  If Aristotle believed in his own theory, then it's probably safe to say that he had absolutely no resemblance to his mother!

- **Contemporary Concepts**

  We still have much to learn. But the proof that you understand how something works is knowing how to fix it when broken: We've come a long way in not only understanding reproduction and fertility, but diagnosing and actually correcting infertility.

So let's talk about your own reproductive motor, how it works, and why it might or might not need a mechanic.

- **Two Roles**

  The male reproductive system does essentially two things. It:

  - *Creates* male genome carrier cells (sperm) within the testes;
  - *Delivers* these carrier cells to the female reproductive tract
    - Delivery happens with the help of:
      - glandular secretions that *feed and protect* the semen
      - muscular contractions that *propel* the semen, and
      - anatomical organs, such as the penis, that *deposit* the semen (inside the female reproductive system)

- **Two Organs**

  The anatomically obvious parts of the male reproductive system are actually sperm *creation* and *delivery* organs:

  - *Scrotum*

    Hanging sack of skin beneath your penis, houses the testicles, or testes, which *create* the sperm cells.

  - *Penis*

    Penetrates the female during sexual intercourse, and acts as the male system's primary sperm *delivery* organ.

- **Sperm Factory**

  Anatomically, the two testes are approximately equal in size (2 x 3/4 x 1 1/4 inches).

  Each testicle houses germ cells ("spermatogonia") which divide and mature through a series of complex biological processes ("spermatogenesis"), eventually leading to the development of mature sperm (see Figure 2). The so-called spermatogonia constantly replenish themselves during the cell division process, so a man can continually produce sperm well into old age.

The entire spermatogenetic process, cell division and maturation from original germ cell to mature sperm, requires about 70 days. On average, you will create over 50 million sperm cells daily for the rest of your life, constantly repeating this little-over-two-month cycle from spermatogonian to mature sperm cell.

FIGURE 1: REPRESENTATION OF THE MALE REPRODUCTIVE SYSTEM

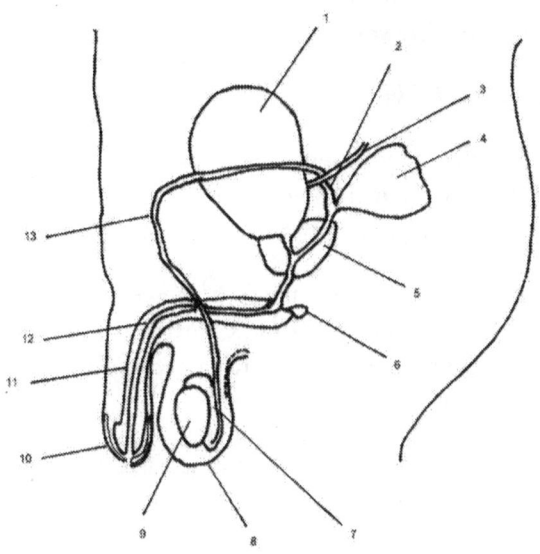

1—Urinary Bladder; 2—Ampulla; 3—Ureter; 4—Seminal Vesicle;
5—Protate; 6—Bulbourethral Gland; 7—Epididymis; 8—Scrotum;
9—Testis; 10—Glans Penis; 11—Urethra; 12—Corpus Cavernosum;
13—Vas Deferens

- **Too Hot To Handle**

  Sperm are finicky about their environment. For sperm to be created and sustained, their ambient temperature must be at least four degrees lower than standard body temperature. Such a need to stay cooler than your average body temperature explains why your testes hang in a sack *outside* your body.

  Sperm are so finicky, in fact, that any increase in temperature caused by, say, working in a very hot environment or having a high fever, will interfere or even destroy sperm production and maintenance. People suffering from a high fever, for instance, will experience a marked drop in sperm count and quality roughly two months after their high temperature breaks. Such a time lag happens since spermatogenesis takes about that long to create new sperm cells.

If for whatever reason you were exposed to these conditions, either externally in the form of extremely hot weather conditions, or internally in the form of fever, you should report this to your fertility physician. Since the resulting detriment to sperm quality is typically temporary, conducting another semen analysis at some point in the future might help improve overall sperm quality and generally re-normalize your results.

"What does a sperm look like?"

The *spermatozoa* (usually called, simply for convenience sake, "sperm") is a tiny cell all of about 1/500th of an inch long and consists of a *head* and *tail* (Figure 2). The head is oval in shape, tapering towards the tip, just like a spear head.

The sperm nucleus makes up approximately 65 percent of the head and consists of genetic material (mostly DNA). The back portion of the head is covered by a sac-like structure that contains enzymes which act something like a chemical warhead, helping the sperm to penetrate the egg.

The tail is about 10 times the length of the head. The initial portion of the tail produces the energy needed for sperm movement, which results from back-and-forth undulations of the tale.

FIGURE 2: REPRESENTATION OF THE HUMAN SPERMATOZOON

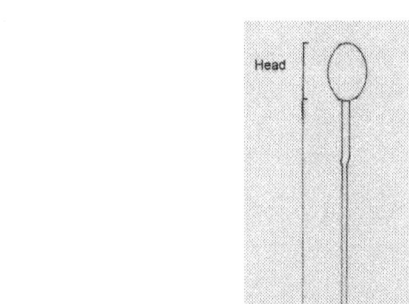

"How many sperm does a man usually produce?"

On average, a man produces about 50 million sperm a day (or about 500 sperm cells per second!). Of these, there are more useless sperm than good sperm, probably due to sloppy workmanship and poor quality control in the testis (not surprising, though, given the tremendous overall volume of production): After all, only a fraction of the sperm produced are actually released during procreation. And of these, some sperm might play a role not directly involved with fertilization.

In essence, Nature retains no practical reason to be exceptionally careful given such mass production activity. Ultimately, "quantity over quality" is Nature's motto when it comes to male reproduction in general and sperm production in particular.

Such a credo is virtually opposite for the female system, which typically creates, protects and must solely rely on but a *single* reproductive cell per month!

"What happnes after sperm creation?"

Sperm are transported from the testes in your scrotum, through the male reproductive system, out and into the female reproductive system along a complex pathway.

Perhaps the best way to understand the entire journey is to describe the various "stations" along the route:

- *Testes*

  As already summarized, sperm are created here through the Spermatogenetic Process. Sperm then leave by way of the *epididymis*, a single, highly convoluted glandular duct that, if you would unwind it, would exceed six meters in length.

- *Epdidymis*

  Anatomically, the epididymis is divided into head, body and tail components. Sperm cells travel from the testes into the attached epididymal head, and then work their way through the body, where various chemical and morphological changes happen to the sperm.

  Epididymal fluids are also added to the sperm, creating the beginning of seminal fluid. Sperm travel slowly through the epididymis, and are subsequently stored in the epididymal tail. The enhanced sperm, contained now in the fluid, are stored here until ejaculation.

- *Vas deferens*

  The epididymal tail leads into the *vas deferens*, a tube approximately 15 inches in total length. During ejaculation, sperm and fluid stored in the epididymis are carried into the vas deferens.

  When sperm reach the end of the vas, additional seminal components are added to the mix from the *accessory sex glands*. The vas deferens joins with the urethra; the sperm end their journey through the male reproductive system via the *penis*.

- *Sex glands*

  These are comprised of the seminal vesicles, the ampulla of the vas deferens, the prostate gland and the bulbourethral (Cowper's) gland. Each gland creates various components that, when taken in total, comprise the *semen*.

And here's some general information: to further describe this complex process:

- *Accessorized*

  Of these glands, the *prostate*, as a result of location and unique glandular architecture, is most prone to infection and cancer. Most physicians highly recommend that all men over the age of 40 should have their prostrates checked on an annual or semi-annual basis, since recovery rates markedly increase based on the relative rapidity of early detection.

- *Ingredients*

  The *seminal vesicles* alone contribute approximately 75 percent to overall ejaculate volume. The prostate provides another 20 percent; all other secretions plus the sperm cells themselves making up the remaining 5 percent.

- *Plasma*

  The fluids from these glands are collectively called the *seminal plasma* of the ejaculate. This seminal plasma provides sperm nourishment and transport. The plasma also contains antibacterial and immune suppressive factors, which ward off infection and protect the sperm.

  Even more importantly, semen helps protect the sperm as they enter the female reproductive system, which can contain contaminants and sperm-debilitating agents in the vaginal mucous. Such natural born agents in the semen enable as many sperm as possible to physically make it to the female egg, or *oocyte*.

- *Swimming Upstream*

  Of the millions upon millions of spermatozoa ejaculated into the vagina during a standard male ejaculation, less than one percent actually reach the uterus. Of these, only one to five thousand spermatozoa are actually able to make it to the fertilization site. One may or may not successfully fertilize the egg, an action dependent on many variables, sheer chance being the primary one.

All excess spermatozoa die and disintegrate, or are more actively removed from the female reproductive system by white blood cells. Some actually leave the tract by passing into the abdominal cavity.

- *No Hurry*

  Interestingly enough, few spermatozoa reach the fertilization site within five to fifteen minutes following insemination: A majority of sperm enter into what's called a "sperm reservoir," where they remain alive for as long as 48 hours or more. During this extended period following intercourse, sperm are gradually released, capable of fertilizing your partner's egg days after coitus.

- *Limited Capacity*

  Sperm, even though fully mature, cannot fertilize an egg until certain membrane alterations (called "capacitation") take place on the sperm surface, induced by the female reproductive tract itself.

  In other words, you may produce *potentially* fertile sperm, but your partner actually renders your sperm fully fertile within her own reproductive system. Significantly, once the egg is actually fertilized, the egg automatically seals her boundary layers, preventing any additional sperm from penetrating.

"Does a man produce male or female sperm?"

- **But of course...**

  Most people, if asked, would conclude that all sperm are, by definition, male (in the sense of containing exclusively male genetic material). After all, the female oocyte, or egg, contains exclusively female genetic material, so what would be the sense or practical point of having a *female sperm*?

  Given a bit of consideration, however, and knowing that, since eggs are exclusively "female" in their genes (being female is therefore the official "default sex" for all human beings), the truth becomes obvious:

- **World Without Women**

  If a couple's offspring contains half the genetic material of the father and half of the mother, then a man must produce an equal number of male sperm *and female sperm*, or females would rapidly become quite rare.

Specifically, the daily result of spermatogenesis is the creation of millions of sperm cells in the testes, half of which contain coding for a female child, half for a male.

- **In Detail**

   In more detail, then, the germ cell, with a full complement of chromosomes (designated "46XY"), divides and gives rise to an equal number of sperm, each with half the amount of chromosomes: Half of them with the male "Y" chromosome (23Y), and half of them with the female "X" chromosome (23X).

   Conversely, the egg contains but one half the complement (23X) of chromosomes. If a sperm with its X chromosome ("female sperm") fertilizes the egg, then the resulting child will be a girl (23X+23X=46XX). If a sperm with its distinctive Y chromosome ("male sperm")fertilizes the egg, then the resulting child will be a boy (23X+23Y=46XY).

"What Happens When I Ejaculate?"

Ejaculation might seem like a fairly straighforward, spontaneous biological process. In actuality, though, the process is highly complex, and involves numerous discrete steps, occuring in sequence.

In general, ejaculation can be characterized as:

- **Obvious**

   Ejaculation is the discharge of semen from the penis. The ejaculatory event consists of external sphincter relaxation, followed by rhythmic contractions.

- **Not So Obvious**

   Prostatic fluid is the first ejaculate component, followed by the sperm-rich fraction from the ampulla and vas deferens. Finally, the seminal vesicular fluid is deposited into the urethra.

   Long story longer, sperm are supplied by nature with everything they need to survive long enough to reach their goal, namely, the egg within your partner's fallopian tube.

   During emission, your bladder neck and external urethral sphincter are closed to contain the deposited seminal fluid. Physical closure of the bladder neck is essential for the prevention of semen flow back into the bladder.

• **Retrograde Motion**

Cutting off the flow to and from your bladder during ejaculation is vital. For some men, this function is impaired or destroyed, resulting in what's called Retrograde Semen Flow. Such flow is detectable with a semen analysis, and correctable through various clinical procedures.

"Billion Dollar Baby"

An elderly man with a substantial fortune decides he would like an heir. Inspired to procreate, he goes for a semen analysis at the local clinic.

When the times comes to collect his sample, he ambles into the collection room and gives it his best shot.

After many minutes, the clinician knocks. "How are you doing, sir?" she asks.

"Oh," the ancient tycoon responds. "I think I could use a little help in here."

Undaunted, the clinican opens the collection room door and enters. She finds the fellow is indeed experiencing some difficulties.

"Are you having trouble ejaculating?" she inquires.

"Ejaculating! I'm having enough trouble just getting the lid off the collection jar!"

"Does the way I collect my semen potentially influence the results?"

Semen collection through masturbation is the most recommended method. Contamination is less likely than through most other methods, and all of your ejaculate can be collected (little, if any, is lost during this procurement process, as opposed to a few of the others we'll talk about).

Ideally, you should produce your semen sample in your physician's office or clinic. Your sample can then almost immediately be analyzed. And since semen quality deteriorates in proportion to length of time following ejaculation, "the sooner the better" applies quite accurately to testing any semen sample.

If producing a sample in your physician's office or clinic is impractical or uncomfortable for you, then a realistic and acceptable alternative is home procurement.

Optimally, stopping by your physician's office and picking up a sterile and seal-able *sample collection container* is a very good idea. Such containers are specifically engineered and designed to safely store your semen, and very good for use when transporting to the lab.

If you must use a household container, try to find a perfectly clean small plastic cup or similar container. If you have to clean the container before use, make sure you do not use any kind of harsh soaps or detergents, since these can leave a resi-due or film on the container, potentially damaging your sperm and reducing overall semen quality.

Another good idea is to line the inside of the collection container with a layer of thin plastic, such as commercially available sandwich bags, etc.

- **Special Methods**

  - *Seminal Pouch*

    If masturbation is not an option for you for whichever reason, be sure and ask your physician about the availability and practice of the seminal pouch collection method. Here, a special condom is used to collect your sperm during coitus. The sample can then be delivered to your doctor for analysis.

  - *Additional Means*

    Impotence due to psychosomatic or medical reasons (such as diabetes or spinal cord injuries) obviously makes masturbation impractical or impossi-ble. In such instances, the use of drugs such as Viagara prior to masturba-tion is often recommended. For other cases, special laboratory methods are required for sperm procurement, including vibratory or electro-stimulation techniques.

- **Non-recommended methods**

  - *Coitus interruptus*

    Commonly called "withdrawal," this method where contamination from vaginal fluid and the loss of initial sperm rich semen are both possible. For similar reasons, oral semen collection and vaginal drainage collection are not recommended.

"How Many Samples Should Be Analyzed?"

As mentioned, large variations in semen quality can occur even between consecutive ejaculates from the same person. Therefore, several ejaculates need to be analyzed to obtain more generalized information about your overall sperm quality. For best results, ejaculates should be analyzed every two or three weeks until a total of four ejaculates have been studied. Only then can an accurate statistical assessment be made of your sperm and its ferlilization capacity.

For practical reasons and general convenience, most folks opt for a simpler procedure: The procurement of at least two ejaculates, analyzed one month apart. If either one of these two ejaculates shows abnormalities, additional ejaculates should then be studied to help confirm the results and narrow down the diagnosis. Then, various methods for sperm enhancement can be considered and eventually implemented to help correct the problem.

Semen quality varies over time, sometimes for the better, other times for the worse. Consequently, all fertility patients should routinely monitor their semen quality at least once or twice each year, for the length of the entire treatment.

"The Sperm Club"

One morning, three men were sitting in the reception area of the fertility clinic, waiting to collect for their semen analyses.

"Smith!" called the receptionist, as the tallest among them went inside.

The other two waited, and waited. Almost an hour later, the tall man finally exited, making room for the next patient.

By sheer coincidence, the following week these same two men found themselves waiting in the reception area. As they recognized each other, the one leaned over and whispered: "Is HE here today, too?"

To which the other replied: "I don't know. But if he is, I hope he spent the week practicing."

"Does Duration Of Sexual Abstinence Affect Semen Quality?"

Literally, many tens of millions of sperm cells are released every time you ejaculate. As a result, sexual abstinence can profoundly influence your semen quality, and therefore the outcome of your semen analysis results. Abstinence is actually one of the most important factors responsible for sperm quality variation.

Make sure to provide your semen sample after the standard abstinence period of at *least* two or three days, since semen analysis standards are established based on this time frame. If you haven't abstained for at least 48 to 72 hours, don't hesitate to reschedule your appointment. And if you don't have an opportunity to reschedule, make sure to inform your doctor exactly how long you have abstained—Your doctor can then adjust his interpretation accordingly.

Some laboratories, in addition to procuring such "optimal" semen samples, also like to obtain a realistic assessment of: "typical" or everyday semen quality: This entails measuring your semen quality after a period of abstinence corresponding to your usual rate of coital frequency. Based on these results, certain behavioral modifications might be suggested to help optimize overall semen quality and thereby increase the likelihood of fertilization.

"No Pain, No Gain"

A young man was counseled as to proper semen analysis procedure. When informed that the required period for sexual abstinence was at least 48 hours, he shouted: "Two days?! How can anybody wait that long?"

An older gentleman, sitting in the waiting room, couldn't help but overhear the outburst, and quipped: "At my age, sonny, I need at least that long before I can get interested in my own hand."

"Where should the Ejaculate Be Collected?"

Preferably, your ejaculate should be collected directly at the laboratory, so that an analysis can be conducted as rapidly as possible to prevent sperm deterioration over time.

If such a method proves impractical, your sample can be hand-delivered to the laboratory, so long as it arrives within twenty minutes. Any amount of time exceeding one hour is strongly ill advised, given the potential damage such lengthy exposure can cause your sperm.

Remember, sperm are finicky about their environment. Your specimen should therefore be protected from temperature extremes during delivery. To maintain a suitable temperature when the weather is cold, for example, the specimen should be kept as close to your body as possible (the inside pocket of a jacket is preferable, say, to simply holding the container in your hand) during transportation to the laboratory. Should the weather prove particularly warm and humid, your sample should be allowed to "breath," while avoiding exposure to direct sunlight. In general, exposure to the elements, too warm or too cold, should be minimized.

Ideally, samples should be collected and analyzed in the laboratory, to prevent any damage, careless or accidental, to your sample. Should any portion of your sample be spilled or in any way lost during delivery, make sure to inform your physician, since such loss can significantly affect your results.

"Parking Permit"

A couple, Harold and Claudia, arrived at the fertility clinic for Harold's semen analysis. When it came time to do the collection, Claudia asked the receptionist if she could join her partner in the collection room.

"I'm afraid that's against our laboratory's policy," the receptionist politely replied.

After some thought, Claudia said: "We'll be right back…"

Minutes later, the couple were in the back seat of their car, doing their best in the parking lot. After several minutes, Claudia exclaimed: "Hurry up, Harold! I don't want to feed the meter again!"

"Do Situation Circumstance And Mood Influence My Semen Quality?"

Very much so. Studies have demonstrated that particularly satisfactory and "enthusiastic" sexual stimulation yields better ejaculate quality than that obtained through masturbation alone. Similarly, any discomfort or even anxiety associated with semen procurement in a clinical setting can affect the volume and overall quality of semen collected.

In other words, the more sustained, satisfying and emotionally significant the sexual response, the higher your resulting semen quality. The relatively sterile settings of a typical laboratory might prove intimidating to many people. Therefore, try to make yourself as comfortable as possible.

After repeat collections, your mind and body should become more accustomed to the procedure. Eventually, with some patience, your relative comfort levels will increase and your anxieties diminish, often reflected by proportionate improvements in your semen analysis results.

"Hard To Please"

A husband and wife were both ushered into their clinic's collection room one morning. After several minutes, the clinic staff heard a disturbance inside, and a clinican knocked on the door.

"Are you guys OK?" the clinican asked.

The shouting seemed to continue, so the clinican slowly opened the door, only to discover the man's wife berating him with gusto.

"Is that all?" she asked, gesturing to the collection container. "Is *that* all you can do?"

"Put yourself in my shoes," explained her husband. "I'm doing my best, honey. You expect me to fill the whole cup?"

"For the amount of money this test is costing me, you'd better!"

Semen Analysis: The Process

"What does a 'semen analysis' actually consist of?"

Semen analysis involves several procedures. The basic procedure is simply called **Routine Semen Analysis (RSA)**. Routine Semen Analysis includes both Gross (Macroscopic) and Microscopic evaluation.

- *Gross Determination*

  Determines semen appearance, coagulation and liquefaction time, viscosity, color, and volume

- *Microscopic Determination*

  Determines sperm concentration, motility, and morphology. The presence of leucocytes and sperm agglutination are also determined.

"Are there other tests available, too?"

Yes. These are called **Specialized Semen Analyses**. They test for such things as sperm ability to migrate into the cervical mucus, sperm membrane integrity, sperm acrosome reaction, sperm zona binding, and sperm penetration assay. In addition, immunological tests to determine the presence of antibodies, and chemical analysis of your seminal plasma are generally available, should the need for them arise.

"Which questions does a Routine Semen Analysis answer?"

- **What does semen look like?**

  Semen is characteristically turbid in appearance. Sperm presence in the seminal fluid makes the semen appear turbid and is used as a very rough estimate of sperm concentration.

  However, contrary to what most might expect: *Semen appearance is of no clinical value in the analysis of human ejaculate.*

- **What happens to semen over time?**

  Immediately following ejaculation, semen normally *coagulates* into a gelatinous mass and then liquefies within thirty minutes when at room temperature, or within fifteen to twenty minutes at 98^0 Fahrenheit.

  The lack (absence) of coagulation may indicate ejaculatory duct obstruction or absence of the seminal vesicles. If your ejaculate has not liquefied after 120 minutes, the sample is abnormal.

  The gynecologist or the reproductive endocrinologist may then recommend IUI or IVF.

- **What should semen usually look like?**

  Semen is usually whitish-grey, pearl white or a yellowish opalescent fluid.

  A reddish color is usually due to red blood cells that are present in the sample, a condition called "hematospermia."

  Urine contamination of your ejaculate may also change semen color and odor. Drugs like methylene blue and pyridium may also change semen color.

  However, again contrary to what you might expect: *Semen color has no significance in the evaluation of fertility.*

- **What is "viscosity"?**

  Viscosity in semen is measured by the "threadiness," or how easily the semen is able to flow.

  The relationship between viscosity and fertility is unknown. High viscosity, however, combined with poor sperm motility, can lead to fertility problems.

  The gynecologist or the reproductive endocrinologist may recommend IUI or IVF.

- **How is semen volume measured?**

  Volume is measured in milliliters and typically measures about half a teaspoon (ranges from two to four milliliters).

  - *Aspermia*

    If you produce no semen at all after orgasm. Aspermia may be due to a clinical problem such as "Retrograde Flow of Semen," Any voided urine following masturbation must be evaluated immediately. If sperm are present, then retrograde semen flow back into the bladder has occurred.

- *Hypospermia*

  If you produce less than 0.5 milliliter of semen (low volume). *Hypospermia* may be due to procedural causes such as an incomplete collection (partially missing the jar), spillage following sample collection, or partial ejaculation due to incomplete orgasm (probably brought about by anxiety, stress, disapproval and embarrassment about masturbation, etc.)

  Hypospermia may also be due to clinical factors which include but are not limited to ejaculatory duct obstruction or absence of the seminal vesicles, to obstruction or stricture of the seminal vesicular duct, inflammation or hypoandrogenism. Consultation with a urologist is recommended.

- *Hyperspermia*

  If you produce more than 6.0 milliliters (high volume). *Hyperspermia* is due to either a long period of sexual abstinence or accessory sex gland fluid overproduction.

  The gynecologist or the reproductive endocrinologist may recommend IUI. The primary physician may also recommend a urologist be consulted.

"A Chip Off The Old Block"

A man was accompanied by his nine-year-old son during his visit to the fertility clinic. They sat waiting patiently along with a waiting room full of other men. At the designated time, the man was called in for his collection.

Less than five minutes later, the man returned to the still crowded waiting room. "OK, kid, let's go!"

The waiting room crowd smirked as his son responded: "Wow, dad. *That* sure was quick!"

- **What is the relationship between semen volume and fertility?**

Overall semen volume has a minimal effect on sperm fertilizing potential, but does aid in the identification of the etiology for the abnormal semen. Low and high semen volumes often lead to subfertility since sperm have difficulty reaching the uterus: Low volumes have trouble reaching the cervix, while relatively high volumes may dilute the overall sperm concentration.

- **What does "Retrograde Flow" mean?**

  Semen flows backwards into the urinary bladder during orgasm. If the patient is aspermic, the initial fraction of the voided urine following a "dry" ejaculation should be checked for sperm. If sperm are indeed present, retrograde flow must have occurred.

  Such retrograde semen flow can be caused by extensive pelvic surgery, lymphadenectomy, sympathectomany, diabetic visceral neuropathy or antihypertensive drugs that block sympathetic tone.

  In these cases, voided urine should be collected immediately following orgasm and checked for sperm. If sperm are present, they should be analyzed for sperm quality.

  The gynecologist or the reproductive endocrinologist may recommend collection of post masturbated urine into a container with sperm media and then process for IUI. The primary physician may also recommend a urologist be consulted.

"What does 'Microscopic Analysis' consist of?"

Cellular elements such as leukocytes, erythrocytes, epithelial cells and bacteria may be present in your seminal fluid.

- **What is "Leukocytospermia"?**

  The presence of a high number of leucocytes (white blood cells) in the seminal fluid and usually assessed as the number of leucocytes per (400 X) high-power field.

  Moderate to heavy amounts (more than five leucocytes per high-power field) of leucocytes present along with seminal debris may suggest a possible accessory sex glands infection. Such infection is likely to affect sperm motility.

  The relationship between leukocyte number and the presence of genital tract infection is unclear. Similarly, the relationship between leukocytes and fertility is unsure. Many gynecologists and reproductive endocrinologists assessing these results might consider leukocytospermia to be a partial factor, rather than a primary cause. The primary physician may also recommend a urologist be consulted.

If the leukocyte count is very high, the ejaculate may appear yellowish-opaque. The condition is sometimes referred to as *pyospermia*. In such cases, a urologist should be consulted. The urologist may recommend semen cultures with a prostatic massage. Antibiotic treatment may be indicated. Occasionally, the apparent leukocytes are really immature sperm and a special stain should be used to correctly distinguish the two.

- **What is "Hematospermia"?**

The presence of fresh or altered blood (red blood cells or erythrocytes) in the ejaculate. Your semen would appear either pinkish or reddish.

Hematospermia may be the result of inflammation, ductal obstruction or cysts, neoplasms, vascular abnormalities, systemic or iatrogenic factors.

Presence of erythrocytes does not appear to influence the absolute fertilizing potential of the sperm. For medical reasons, the gynecologist or primary physician may recommend that a urologist be consulted.

"Blood Simple"

A fairly young, robust-looking man went for a routine semen analysis. Ushered into the collection room, everything seemed to be smooth sailing. But the staff waited. And waited.

Finally, after close to an hour, the nurse politely knocked on the door. "Excuse me, sir. But are you all right?"

The man opened the door, and sat back down inside.

The nurse entered, and asked again: "Are you OK?"

To which the man responded, somewhat impatiently: "Aren't you going to take my blood first?"

- **What are epithelial cells?**

Some epithelial cells, possibly originating from the urethra or from the meatus and glands are contaminants occurring during masturbation. They are commonly present in your seminal fluid and are typically of no significance.

Many epithelial cells within the sample may indicate that collection was by coitus interruptus, or orally. These semen collection methods may sometimes compromise the sperm quantity and quality.

- **What about microorganisms?**

Microorganisms may be found in your ejaculate.

The gynecologist or primary physician may regard them as either *commensals* or *contaminants*. Large numbers of such organisms may indicate a genital tract infection.

The gynecologist or primary physician may recommend that a urologist be consulted.

- **What about cells of "Spermatogenic Origin"?**

These are the precursors of sperm cells, or essentially, immature sperm cells.

The presence of these cells in relatively high concentration is usually associated with below normal sperm count and abnormal sperm morphology. This finding may suggest an overall reduction in fertility potential.

In acute distress situations (such as fever, intoxications, exposure to radiation or cytotoxic drugs), an abnormal number of sperm precursors may be present in the ejaculate, prior to the patient becoming azoospermic.

The gynecologist or primary physician may recommend a repeat analysis to confirm the presence of these precursors. If confirmed, a urological consultation may be suggested.

- **What is Sperm Agglutination?**

"Sperm agglutination" is sperm clumping into aggregates. Agglutination encompasses two types of clumping: *Non-Specific* and *Site-Specific*.

- Non-specific agglutination

  Sperm cells adhere to various seminal debris, leucocytes or mucous threads, and various other non-sperm cellular elements.

  Non-specific agglutination, depending on how extensive, might suggest an accessory sex gland infection. However, merely a few clusters of immotile agglutinated sperm clinging to debris, mucus, and the like is of no clinical significance.

- Site-specific agglutination: Sperm cells adhere to each other in a site-specific manner, such as head-to-head, head-to-tail, tail-to-tail, or any combination like that.

  Site-specific agglutination typically signifies an immunological cause (*see: Antisperm Antibody Tests*).

When sperm agglutination is high, the physician may recommend an anti-sperm antibody test and may also recommend a urologist be consulted.

- **What are "Sperm Concentration" and "Sperm Count"?**

Sperm concentration is the number of sperm per milliliter of semen. Sperm count is the total number of sperm per ejaculate.

- *Azoospermia*

  If you produce no sperm in the ejaculate. Azoospermia diagnosis should be made only after an undiluted ejaculate is centrifuged, and the complete absence of spermatozoa in the centrifuge pellet is microscopically confirmed in not less than two different ejaculates. Azoospermia is divided into obstructive type and non-obstructive type.

  Azoospermia may be due to hormonal insufficiency, congenital factors, ejaculatory duct obstruction, therapeutic, and immunological factors. Idiopathic and genetic factors may also be involved.

- *Oligozoospermia*

  If you produce less than 20.0×10^6 sperm per milliliter by World Health Organization Standard. Some laboratories now set this value at 10.0×10^6 or even as low as 5×10^6 sperm per milliliter (low sperm count).

  Oligozoospermia may be due to procedural causes (initial semen fraction loss during collection), clinical factors (such as partial obstruction, hyperprolactemia, varicocele, cryptorchidism, diabetes mellitus and multiple sclerosis), and therapeutic factors. Idiopathic and genetic factors may also be involved.

  Azoospermia *or* Oligozoospermia may be due to thermal stress (acute high fever), congenital factors (about 12 percent of azoospermic men and about 7 percent of severely oligozoospermic men have microdeletions in their Y-Chromosome).

It can also be due to therapeutic factors, habitual factors (chronic alcoholism, nicotine, marijuana, and morphine), or even environmental pollutants.

- *Polyzoospermia*

  If you produce more than 250 x 10^6 sperm per milliliter (high sperm count).

  Polyzoospermia is usually due to long periods of sexual abstinence. Relatively high sperm concentrations of 700.0 x 10^6 sperm per milliliter or more usually result in poor overall sperm quality. Fertility potential may also be compromised.

- **Is Sperm Count alone an indicator of fertility?**

Sperm count alone, although a potentially determining factor, is *not* an accurate indicator of fertilizing potential.

The determination of low fertility potential, based solely upon sperm count, is extremely uncertain. As long as a single sperm is present in the ejaculate, the possibility for fertilization, however remote, nonetheless exists. Thus, below average sperm production is compatible with fertility so long as overall sperm quality remains acceptable and no problems exist with the spouse's reproductive status. However, to hasten fertility treatment outcome, your physician may recommend IUI, IVF or even IVF with ICSI.

Sᴘᴇʀᴍ Oɴ Pᴀʀᴀᴅᴇ: Tʜᴇ Cᴏᴜɴᴛ

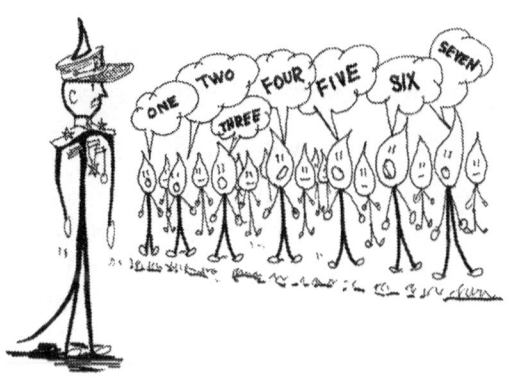

- **What about temperature? How does that affect my fertility?**

Sperm production is dependent on testicular temperature. Ambient temperature, even though relatively high, should not affect spermatogenesis (if temperature remains within a tolerable range).

The human body's ability to thermoregulate core body temperature should provide an adequate compensatory effect. However, occupational exposure (such as a furnace or boiler room, the work-related thermal variation of fire fighters, professional cooks, truck and taxi drivers etc.) may produce thermal stress sufficient for the reduction of semen quality.

Please note that such factors as tight fitting underwear, saunas, prolonged immersion in hot water (whirlpool) baths and steam (Turkish) baths do not seem to have the debilitating effects once thought. However, the physician may recommend avoiding these, at least during the course of infertility treatment.

- **What are the differences between azoospermia and oligozoospermia?**

The differentiation between azoospermia and oligozoospermia is important clinically because respective therapeutic recommendations can vary greatly.

Repeat analysis is a must, prior to definitive diagnosis.

The gynecologist or the reproductive endocrinologist may recommend IUI, IVF and may also suggest a urologist be consulted. As a viable alternative, the physician may recommend artificial insemination with donor sperm.

- **What is "Sperm Motility"?**

The percent sperm motility is the ratio of motile (moving) sperm number to total sperm number and is expressed as a percentage.

- *Asthenozoospermic* (low sperm motility percentage)

  If sperm in your ejaculate is less than 50 percent motile by World Health Organization Standard. If all spermatozoa are immotile, the condition is referred to as *necrozoospermia*. A rare disorder exists where the sperm are immotile but viable and a vital stain test will distinguish between viable and dead sperm.

Asthenozoospermia may be due to procedural causes (psychological, physiological and methodological), congenital factors, clinical factors, immunological factors or idiopathic factors.

- **What is the relationship between motility and fertility?**

Abnormal sperm (except for headless or pin-point sperm) never show good motility, so good motility is therefore an inherent characteristic of good sperm. However, one should be aware that a sperm with abnormal DNA may look and behave like normal sperm, yet exhibit zero fertility potential.

As a general rule, it could be stated that *all fertile sperm are naturally motile* but *not all motile sperm are naturally fertile*. For example, all kings are men but not all men are kings.

SUPER-MOTILE RACING SPERM

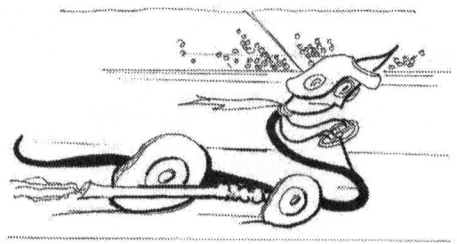

- **What is "Progressive Sperm Motility"?**

Progressive sperm motility is a percentage of the number of motile sperm moving in a linear, forward moving, direction. Usually, *progressive* sperm motility should be 75 percent or more of the *overall* sperm motility.

Motility is only one of many variables influencing fertility; consequently, sperm motility must be extremely low to actually be the sole infertility cause. Because dead or poorly motile spermatozoa affect fertilizing capacity of other sperm, removal of these sperm is useful prior to IUI or IVF.

The gynecologist or reproductive endocrinologist depending on the severity of asthenozoospermia, may recommend techniques to separate motile from immotile sperm prior to IUI, IVF. They may also suggest a urologist be consulted.

- **What is "Sperm Morphology"?**

Sperm shape and appearance of your sperm.

A semen smear is prepared on a slide, air dried, fixed, stained and examined at a 1000 X magnification. Microscopic evaluations are subjective, and interpretations of abnormality vary according to the observer. More than 70 different morphological abnormalities have been identified.

- *Teratozoospermic* (low normal sperm morphology percentage)

  If sperm in your ejaculate displays more than 70 percent abnormal morphology by World Health Organization Standard. Generally, these can be grouped according to abnormalities of the head, mid piece, tail, tapered forms, or combinations thereof (amorphous forms) and sperm precursors.

  Teratozoospermia may be due to clinical factors (Fever, Varicocele, Allergic Reactions), therapeutic factors, stress factors, or congenital factors.

  A particular diagnosis is justified when specific sperm abnormalities are demonstrated to occur frequently in the ejaculate, not just occasionally.

- **Are there usually a high percentage of abnormal sperm in semen?**

A relatively high number of abnormal sperm forms are present in normal human semen. Although 70 percent abnormal sperm morphology indicates a testicular or epididymal impairment, *fertility potential need not be compromised.*

Morphological abnormalities must be extremely high in semen for fertility to be affected. Therefore, repeat analysis is recommended, prior to definitive diagnosis.

The gynecologist or the reproductive endocrinologist depending on the percentage of abnormal sperm morphology, may recommend IUI, IVF, or IVF with ICSI. They may also suggest a urologist be consulted.

As a viable alternative, the physician may recommend artificial insemination with donor sperm.

"When should a 'Specialized Semen Analysis' be performed?"

When Routine Semen Analysis results are either within normal range, or yield equivocal values, specialized tests are then recommended. When the spouse is found to be normal, specialized tests may then be recommended on the male spouse.

Please note that these tests are not routinely performed, and your own physician may or may not have access to them. Consequently, you might be referred to another laboratory capable of performing these specialized tests.

"What do these 'Specialized' Tests consist of?"

Numerous tests are available. These include:

- **Sperm Mucus Penetration Test**

  Spermatozoa may appear normal but may not be able to penetrate and migrate through the cervical mucus and consequently cannot reach the fertilization site. Such migratory capacity or incapacity can be tested by allowing the sperm to penetrate and move through cervical mucus *in vitro*. Failure of *in vitro* penetration is often thought to imply failure *in vivo*.

  Actively motile spermatozoa with good forward progression typically score well in these tests, so this specialized test is predominantly useful with already questionable samples.

Once diagnosis is made, the gynecologist or reproductive endocrinologist may recommend IUI.

- **Sperm Membrane Integrity Test**

  Membrane integrity is important to sperm success. Sperm motility, sperm capacitation, and the binding of sperm to egg surface can all be compromised should membrane integrity prove questionable or in any way inadequate. Thus, sperm membrane integrity and functionality is significant, and membrane function assessment may prove a vital part of overall sperm fertilizing capacity.

  Two tests are available to evaluate spermatozoon membrane integrity: The *Supravital* (viability, live-dead stain) and the *Hypoosmotic Swelling* (HOS) test.

  The supravital stain determines whether the membrane is physically intact or not. When damaged or broken the eosin Y dye is able to stain the sperm; if the membrane is intact, the dye is unable to penetrate the sperm. The stain thus evaluates the viability of a cell through the inclusion or exclusion of the eosin Y dye.

The HOS test determines sperm membrane functional integrity through response to an osmotic stress. The sample is *normal* if the tested sperm shows more than 60 percent reactive ("swollen") sperm; the sample is deemed *abnormal* if fewer than 50 percent of such reactive sperm are present. Non viable sperm will not become "swollen" in this HOS test.

The events that allow sperm to fertilize involve changes in the sperm membrane system (capacitation and acrosome reaction) and are a process that occurs when sperm are in the female reproductive tract. The spermatozoa membrane must be intact and functional for these events to occur.

Once an abnormal diagnosis is made, the gynecologist or reproductive endocrinologist may recommend IUI or IVF. As a viable alternative, the physician may recommend artificial insemination with donor sperm.

- **Hemizona or Zona Binding Test**

  To determine whether sperm capacitation has occurred, sperm can be added to isolated human zona pellucida or to zona free hamster oocytes and the extent of binding or penetration can be determined. If spermatozoa are capacitated, they will undergo the acrosome reaction and bind or penetrate oocytes.

  Such spermatozoon binding activity can be tested by using oocytes from a variety of sources: nonliving, intact human oocytes; isolated zonae obtained from autopsy-derived ovaries, from surgically excised ovarian tissue; or from immature or surplus unfertilized oocytes after IVF. More than 90 percent of the tightly zona bound spermatozoa undergo the acrosome reaction, so that this test can be used to estimate the number of spermatozoa undergoing this reaction.

  Only a few laboratories presently perform the hemizona or zona binding test due to the scarcity of human zona pellucida.

Once an abnormal diagnosis is made, the gynecologist or reproductive endocrinologist may recommend IVF with ICSI. As a viable alternative, the physician may recommend artificial insemination with donor sperm.

- **Sperm Penetration Test**

  Spermatozoa must bind and penetrate the egg vitelline membrane, a prerequisite to fusion with the egg contents. Zona free (denuded) hamster eggs will allow capacitated sperm from other species to bind and penetrate the egg. This capacity is utilized to evaluate ability to bind and penetrate the egg vitelline membrane of human spermatozoa.

Zona-free hamster oocytes are added to capacitated sperm droplets and incubated for two to three hours. Following incubation, the oocytes are examined microscopically for sperm penetration.

The test is useful, but the data need to be interpreted with care and should be considered only in conjunction with the other sperm test results. When no or poor penetration occurs, the test should always be repeated (possibly under different conditions) before reaching a definite conclusion.

Once an abnormal diagnosis is made, the gynecologist or reproductive endocrinologist may repeat the test and recommend IVF with ICSI. As a viable alternative, the physician may recommend artificial insemination with donor sperm.

- **Strict Morphology Determination**

  Meticulous analysis of stained spermatozoa can identify many minor deviations from an otherwise "perfect" sperm cell. If such detailed analysis reveals fewer than 14 percent "normal" sperm, then the sample has abnormal morphology. Such an assessment usually proves valuable for IVF outcome.

  Once diagnosis is made, the gynecologist or reproductive endocrinologist may recommend IVF. Since ICSI is highly effective for sperm with abnormal morphology, IVF with ICSI may prove particularly advantageous.

- **Antisperm Antibody Tests**

  When sperm are exposed to (come into contact with) the immune reacting cells in the circulatory system, the body responds by producing antibodies against spermatozoa. Antisperm antibodies primarily cause sperm agglutination, immobilization or surface binding, and may cause infertility in 12 percent to 20 percent of couples who have no other demonstrable explanations.

  Many different methods are available for evaluation of antisperm antibodies in blood, seminal plasma, spermatozoa, and cervical mucus. Methods that test for serum antisperm antibodies are referred to as indirect tests, while tests for antibodies on patients' spermatozoa are called direct tests.

  Sperm antibodies may interfere with spermatogenesis and sperm maturation in the male, and hinder sperm transport, cervical mucus penetration, capacitation, and fertilization in the female. Antisperm antibodies may also hinder sperm fertilizing capacity.

Much confusion exists regarding antibody test interpretation because a direct correlation between sperm antibodies and infertility does not exist. Antibody presence probably indicates a genital tract disturbance, which may be the primary cause of infertility or subfertility, rather than the antibodies themselves.

At present, prevalent sperm antibodies should be taken as an indication that immunologic problems may exist. In some cases, these antibodies can account for fertility problems, but in other cases, they are only contributory.

Once diagnosis is made, your partner's gynecologist or reproductive endocrinologist may recommend therapy consisting of steroid treatment, IUI, IVF, or IVF with ICSI.

• **Chemical Analysis of Seminal Plasma**

Your prostate, seminal vesicles and epididymis produce components that are quite specific for each gland. These components are probably non-essential for sperm function, so their usefulness as fertility indicators is limited. However, these components help assess accessory sex gland status.

Particular components are produced by a particular gland, such as fructose by the seminal vesicles and zinc by the prostate gland.

Semen pH can be a significant factor in ejaculate analysis. However, semen pH has little direct significance to sperm fertility potential, unless levels are excessively abnormal.

The relative contribution of these chemicals and their evaluation can prove diagnostically useful to identify or confirm male genital tract obstruction.

If seminal plasma chemical composition abnormalities are observed, your partner's gynecologist or physician may recommend consultation with a urologist.

"A whole lot seems to be going on here. Can you simplify and summarize?"

Fertilization involves direct sperm-egg union. Essentially, sperm must be able to reach the fertilization site by possessing adequate *sperm motility* and *sperm morphology*. Sperm must also be present in sufficient numbers within the semen *(sperm concentration)* to overcome the statistical improbabilities of finally reaching the egg. The first obstacle in the female reproductive system is the cervical mucus. Sperm must penetrate and migrate through the cervical mucus (evaluated by a *sperm mucus penetration assay),*

Sperm, during passage through the female reproductive system, must undergo membrane alteration known as sperm capacitation. Once the sperm reach the egg, the spermatozoa must undergo further membrane alteration leading to acrosome reaction, which is dependent on the functional integrity of the membrane itself *(evaluated by a hypoosmotic swelling assay).* Sperm must then bind and penetrate the zona pellucida (evaluated by a *zona binding assay)* prior to fusing with the egg's vitelline membrane (evaluated by a *sperm penetration assay).*

According to the prescribed sperm function outline, male fertility potential can best be evaluated in a similarly logical and sequential manner. Each question involves the successful completion of a vital sperm step of the fertilization process. If that step is hindered in any capacity, then the corresponding tests are available to confirm the diagnosis and thereby hopefully help correct the problem:

- **Are the sperm able to reach the fertilization site?**

   Routine Semen Analysis and *Sperm Mucus Penetration Assay* are tests which enable that determination.

- **Are the sperm able to fertilize an egg?**

   Hypoosmotic Swelling Assay, Zona Binding Assay and *Sperm Penetration Assay* allow that determination in an in vitro environment.

- **Are immunological factors suspected?**

   Antisperm antibodies have been implicated in 10 to 20 percent of unexplained infertility cases. Such a test panel should assess all three effects of antisperm antibodies *(sperm agglutination, sperm immobilization* and *sperm surface binding).*

- **Do chemical components need to be assessed?**

   Yes, based on the results of a routine semen analysis, since a chemical component test will assesses fluid contribution from the epididymis, seminal vesicle, and prostate. The pH level should also be determined.

Please note that none of these tests can evaluate sperm ability to travel through the female reproductive tract, and reach your partner's egg.

"Topsy-Turvy"

Bob asked Jack how his friend's fertility treatment was coming along.

"Oh, all right I guess," responded Jack. "My wife's busy trying to get pregnant, and my hand is hurting from doing all the work."

"Well," replied Bob. "Be thankful it's not the other way around."

Conclusion

The primary purpose of semen analysis is to determine your sperm fertility potential. Ironically enough, although the fertilization process is fairly well understood, the fertilizing capacity of any particular ejaculate is difficult to determine. Your sperm are extremely complex, and can become infertile when any one of a number of highly sensitive biochemical, physiological or morphologic entities is disturbed. Such complexity makes fertilization evaluation particularly difficult when one or several of these attributes deviate only slightly from normal. Of course, an infertile ejaculate can be fairly conclusively identified when one sperm variable is significantly or absolutely abnormal.

Whenever a sperm abnormality is reported, a repeat semen analysis should be performed to confirm the observation. Some abnormalities are even congenital. For example, about 3 percent of men of reproductive age may be azoospermic. Of these men, a signficant percentage are due to microdeletions in their Y-chromosomes. Once the exact nature of the abnormality is confirmed, then the recommendation of the physician handling the fertility treatment should be followed.

So long as you are able to produce mature sperm, techniques are available which can help circumvent the typical fertilization process. These techniques include IUI, IVF and IVF with ICSI. In fact, male fertility treatment has come a long way. Men once considered "sterile" are now able to have children. And if you are unable to ejaculate mature sperm, special techniques, known as Microscopic Epididymal Sperm Aspiration (MESA) and Testicular Sperm Extraction (TESA) are available to obtain sperm directly from your reproductive system. Sperm acquired in this new way can then be used with IVF and ICSI.

Remember that you should never underestimate the importance of your female partner's reproductive status. A vital element of fertility analysis involves consideration of the female reproductive status, and it's relationship with the interacting sperm. Since the primary physician managing an infertile couple is aware of the couples' reproductive situation, he or she should be the one to make the final interpretation and recommendation.

As a general rule, a properly informed and interested patient makes the entire fertility management process easier for himself, his spouse and everyone else involved. If you have any questions not answered by this booklet, don't hesitate to ask your physician!

Hopefully, the explanations provided in this book have helped you to better understand semen analysis and the basic interpretation of semen analysis results.

Terminology

SEMEN VOLUME

- Aspermia
  No semen

- Hypospermia
  Less than 0.5 ml semen

- Hyperspermia
  More than 6.0 ml semen

SPERM CONCENTRATION

- Azoospermia
  No spermatozoa in the seminal fluid

- Oligozoospermia
  Less than 20×10^6 sperm/ml (by WHO Standard)

- Polyzoospermia
  More than 250×10^6 sperm/ml

SPERM QUALITY

- Normozoospermia
  Between 20 and 250×10^6 sperm/ml with more than 40% sperm motility and normal morphology respectively

SPERM MOTILITY

- Asthenozoospermia
  Less than 50% motility (by World Health Organization Standard)

- Necrozoospermia
  Absence of sperm motility

SPERM MORPHOLOGY

* Teratozoospermia
  More than 70% abnormal sperm (by WHO Standard)

* Oligoasthenozoospermia,
  Oligoasthenoteratozoospermia (or other combinations)
  Signify various disturbances among the variables listed above.

Definitions & Acronyms

ARTIFICIAL INSEMINATION *(AI)*

The term artificial insemination was used by fertility specialists to distinguish between intercourse and the laboratory insemination process. The acronym *AI* was assigned to this procedure. Since AI is feasible with spouse or even donor sperm, the acronyms later became *AIH (Artificial Insemination with Husband sperm)* or *AID (Artificial Insemination with Donor sperm)*. After AIDS became recognized as a disease, the term AID obviously lost popularity. Instead, fertility specialists now use the term *TID (Therapeutic Insemination with Donor sperm)*, or *TDI (Therapeutic Donor Insemination)*.

When the semen, contained in a cap, is placed over the cervix, the procedure is referred to as *Pericervical Insemination (CAP Insemination)* or when it is placed inside the cervix, the procedure is referred to as *Intracervical Insemination (ICI)*.

When sperm is isolated from semen and placed into the uterus through the cervix, the procedure is referred to as *IntraUterine Insemination (IUI)*. If sperm is placed inside the fallopian tube (the anterior part of the uterus) the procedure is referred to as *Fallopian Sperm Perfusion (FSP)*.

ASSISTED REPRODUCTIVE TECHNOLOGY *(ART)*

These include procedures to assist infertile couples achieve a pregnancy. ART includes procedures such as *In Vitro Fertilization (IVF), Gamete Intra-Fallopian Transfer (GIFT)* and *Zygote Intra-Fallopian Transfer (ZIFT)*.

In *IVF*, ova (eggs) collected from the female reproductive tract are inseminated with sperm and allowed to fertilize in vitro. The resulting embryos are then transferred back to the patient. The fertilized egg or the embryo converts to a fetus in the uterus and the woman carries the fetus to term. If the fertilized egg (or zygote stage) is transferred back, the term *ZIFT* is used.

If the ova and sperm are transferred to the anterior of the uterus before in vitro fertilization, the term *GIFT* is used.

If a sperm is injected into the egg instead of incubating ova with numerous sperm, then the process is called *Intra-Cytoplasmic Sperm Injection (ICSI)*.

When sperm are micro surgically aspirated from the epididymis for *ICSI*, the process is called *Microscopic Epididymal Sperm Aspiration (MESA)*, and when it is extracted from the testis, the process is called *Testicular Sperm Extraction (TESE)*.

About the Author

R.S. Jeyendran, D.V.M., M.S., Ph.D., HCLD

Dr. Jeyendran is a reproductive physiologist specializing in semen analysis techniques and procedures. He has authored more than 275 scientific articles, reviews, book chapters and abstracts in male reproduction.

He has written three other books. The first, entitled *Interpretation of Semen Analysis Results: A Practical Guide*, remains the only guidebook for the clinical interpretation of semen analysis results published by Cambridge University Press. His *Sperm Collection and Processing Methods* is a procedural anthology is by the same publisher. Dr. Jeyendran's third book, *Protocols for Semen Analysis in Clinical Diagnosis* is published by Parthenon Publishing.

Dr. Jeyendran is presently the Director of Andrology Laboratory Services and a Research Professor in the Department of Physical Medicine and Rehabilitation, Northwestern University Medical School, Chicago.

SPERM A+: RESULTS GET A "THUMBS UP!"

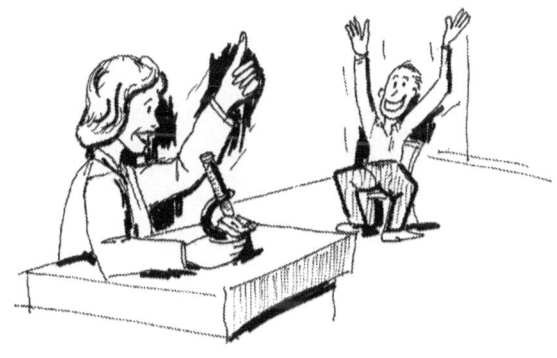

0-595-27964-3

www.ingramcontent.com/pod-product-compliance
Lightning Source LLC
Chambersburg PA
CBHW021036180526
45163CB00005B/2153